Histamine Intolerance

Factors Influencing
Histamine Levels

By

Blair Aonghas

Table of Contents

CHAPTER 1
Introduction

Histamine intolerance is a condition that has gained increasing recognition in recent years as an underlying cause of various chronic and often perplexing health issues. While histamine is a naturally occurring compound in the human body and plays a crucial role in various physiological processes, including immune response and regulating stomach acid, some individuals are unable to tolerate normal levels of histamine due to an imbalance between histamine production and degradation. This imbalance leads to a wide range of symptoms and discomfort, collectively known as histamine intolerance.

1.1 What is Histamine Intolerance

Histamine intolerance, also referred to as histamine sensitivity or histaminosis, is a condition characterized by the body's inability to effectively break down histamine, resulting in an excess of this compound in the bloodstream. Histamine is a biogenic amine that serves as a neurotransmitter and a signaling molecule. It is produced by various cells in the body, particularly mast cells and basophils, and plays a pivotal role in allergic reactions, immune responses, and the regulation of gastric acid.

Individuals with histamine intolerance have a compromised ability to metabolize histamine due to a deficiency or dysfunction of the enzyme diamine oxidase (DAO) or histamine N-methyltransferase (HNMT), both of which are responsible for breaking down histamine. This metabolic impairment leads to histamine accumulating in the body, causing a wide range of symptoms, often resembling allergies or allergic reactions.

1.2 Symptoms and Diagnosis

The symptoms of histamine intolerance can manifest in a diverse array of ways, making it challenging to diagnose. Common symptoms include:

- Gastrointestinal symptoms: These may include abdominal pain, bloating, diarrhea, constipation, and nausea.

- Skin and allergic reactions: Skin issues such as hives, itching, and redness can occur. Additionally, individuals with histamine intolerance may experience nasal congestion, runny nose, sneezing, and itchy or watery eyes.

- Respiratory symptoms: Histamine intolerance can lead to asthma-like symptoms, including coughing and wheezing, as well as difficulty breathing.

- Other systemic symptoms: Individuals with histamine intolerance may experience headaches, migraines, fatigue, irregular heartbeat, and mood disturbances, among other symptoms.

Diagnosing histamine intolerance can be a complex process. Healthcare providers often rely on medical history, symptom assessment, and the exclusion of other conditions with similar symptoms. Specific laboratory tests, including measuring DAO enzyme activity and histamine levels in the blood, can provide supportive evidence of the condition. The gold standard for diagnosis is a controlled elimination diet, where histamine-rich foods and beverages are temporarily removed from the diet, and symptoms are monitored for improvement. Reintroducing these foods can lead to symptom recurrence, further confirming the diagnosis.

1.3 Causes and Triggers

Understanding the causes and triggers of histamine intolerance is critical for managing the condition. While the exact causes are not always clear, several factors are known to contribute:

- **Enzyme Deficiency**: The most common cause of histamine intolerance is a deficiency of the enzymes DAO or HNMT, responsible for breaking down histamine. This deficiency can be due to genetics, underlying medical conditions, or medications that interfere with enzyme function.

- **Gut Health**: The gut plays a pivotal role in histamine metabolism, and imbalances in the gut microbiota can lead to increased histamine production. Conditions like small intestinal bacterial overgrowth (SIBO) and leaky gut can exacerbate histamine intolerance.

- **Dietary Factors**: Certain foods are naturally high in histamine or trigger histamine release within the body. These include aged cheeses, processed and fermented foods, alcohol, and certain fruits and vegetables. Additionally, some individuals may react to foods that block DAO activity or contain histamine-liberating substances.

- **Medications and Supplements**: Certain medications, such as non-steroidal anti-inflammatory drugs (NSAIDs) and antacids, can interfere with histamine degradation or trigger histamine release. In some cases, supplements that contain histamine or histamine-releasing substances can exacerbate symptoms.

- **Stress and Hormonal Factors**: Stress and hormonal fluctuations, especially in women, can influence histamine levels and exacerbate symptoms. Stress management and hormone regulation are crucial aspects of managing histamine intolerance.

Understanding the causes and triggers of histamine intolerance is essential for developing an effective management plan. This often involves dietary modifications, addressing gut health, and, in some cases, the use of medications or supplements to support histamine metabolism. Histamine intolerance is a complex condition, and its management is highly individualized, with a focus on symptom relief and improving the quality of life for those affected.

CHAPTER 2

Understanding Histamine

2.1 The Role of Histamine in the Body

Histamine is a biogenic amine that serves as a crucial signaling molecule in the human body. It plays several essential roles in physiological processes, particularly in the immune system and the gastrointestinal tract. Understanding the multifaceted role of histamine is essential in comprehending how its imbalance can lead to histamine intolerance.

Immune Response: Histamine is released by mast cells and basophils, two types of white blood cells, during an immune response. When the body encounters a pathogen or allergen, histamine is one of the first responders. It helps orchestrate the inflammatory response, which includes dilating blood vessels, increasing vascular permeability, and attracting other immune cells to the site of infection or injury. While these actions are vital for immune defense, excessive or prolonged histamine release can lead to the symptoms of histamine intolerance.

Gastric Acid Regulation: In the stomach, histamine acts as a neurotransmitter to stimulate the production of gastric acid (stomach acid). Specifically, histamine binds to H2 receptors on the stomach lining, triggering the release of acid. This acid is necessary for proper digestion, breaking down food for absorption. However, an overproduction of stomach acid due to an excess of histamine or excessive H2 receptor activation can lead to conditions such as acid reflux and peptic ulcers.

Neurotransmitter: In the nervous system, histamine functions as a neurotransmitter. It plays a role in wakefulness, attention, and cognitive functions. Medications that target histamine receptors in the brain, like antihistamines, can cause drowsiness due to their influence on histaminergic pathways.

2.2 Histamine Metabolism

Histamine metabolism is the process by which the body manages the levels of histamine, ensuring it remains within a balanced range. This is critical for preventing excessive histamine buildup and the onset of histamine intolerance. Two primary enzymes are responsible for histamine metabolism: diamine oxidase (DAO) and histamine N-methyltransferase (HNMT).

- **Diamine Oxidase (DAO)**: DAO is an enzyme found in the lining of the digestive tract, where it primarily degrades histamine from ingested foods. Its role is to break down histamine and convert it into an inactive form. When DAO activity is compromised, histamine from dietary sources can accumulate, contributing to symptoms of histamine intolerance. Factors such as genetics, gut health, and certain medications can affect DAO activity.

- **Histamine N-Methyltransferase (HNMT)**: HNMT is another enzyme responsible for histamine degradation, particularly in the central nervous system. It functions by transferring a methyl group to histamine, converting it into N-methylhistamine. While DAO primarily acts in the gut, HNMT primarily functions in the brain, helping to regulate histamine levels in neural synapses. Genetic variations in HNMT can also influence histamine intolerance.

Histamine metabolism is a dynamic and finely balanced process. When either of these enzymes is compromised or when histamine production exceeds degradation capacity, histamine intolerance can occur. Understanding the intricacies of this metabolic pathway is vital for both diagnosis and management of the condition, as interventions often aim to support these enzymes and reduce histamine levels in the body to alleviate symptoms.

2.3 Factors Influencing Histamine Levels

The levels of histamine in the body are influenced by a complex interplay of various factors, and understanding these factors is crucial in managing histamine intolerance. Here are some of the key factors that can influence histamine levels:

1. **Dietary Intake**: Perhaps the most significant factor affecting histamine levels is the foods and beverages consumed. Certain foods are naturally high in histamine, such as aged cheeses, fermented products (e.g., sauerkraut, yogurt), alcoholic beverages, and processed meats. Histamine-rich foods can directly contribute to an increase in histamine levels in the body, particularly in individuals with histamine intolerance. Additionally, some foods contain histamine-releasing substances, such as tomatoes, eggplants, and spinach, which can exacerbate symptoms.

2. **Enzyme Activity**: The activity of enzymes responsible for

histamine metabolism, especially diamine oxidase (DAO) and histamine N-methyltransferase (HNMT), is a critical factor. Reduced activity of these enzymes due to genetic factors, gastrointestinal conditions, or the use of certain medications can impair histamine degradation, leading to an accumulation of histamine in the body.

3. **Gut Health**: The gut plays a significant role in histamine metabolism. Conditions like small intestinal bacterial overgrowth (SIBO) can lead to increased histamine production in the gut, contributing to histamine intolerance. Leaky gut syndrome, where the intestinal lining becomes more

permeable, can also allow histamine to pass into the bloodstream more easily.

4. **Medications and Supplements**: Certain medications can interfere with histamine metabolism and lead to increased histamine levels. Non-steroidal anti-inflammatory drugs (NSAIDs), proton pump inhibitors (PPIs), and some antidepressants are examples of medications that can impact histamine regulation. In addition, supplements containing histamine or histamine-releasing substances may exacerbate symptoms.

5. **Stress and Hormones**: Stress, both physical and emotional, can influence histamine levels.

During periods of stress, the body may release more histamine as part of the stress response, exacerbating symptoms in individuals with histamine intolerance. Hormonal fluctuations, particularly in women, can also influence histamine levels and symptom severity.

6. **Genetic Factors**: Genetic variations can affect the enzymes responsible for histamine metabolism. Some individuals may inherit genetic mutations that result in reduced DAO or HNMT activity, making them more susceptible to histamine intolerance.

7. **Environmental Allergens**: Exposure to environmental allergens, such as pollen, dust

mites, and pet dander, can trigger the release of histamine in individuals with allergies. This histamine release is a normal part of the body's immune response but can exacerbate histamine intolerance symptoms in sensitive individuals.

8. **Alcohol and Smoking**: Alcohol consumption can lead to increased histamine release in the body and impede histamine metabolism. Smoking also affects histamine regulation and can contribute to histamine intolerance symptoms.

These factors and their interactions is essential for managing histamine intolerance. By identifying and addressing the specific factors that affect an individual, it's possible to develop a tailored approach to reduce histamine levels and alleviate symptoms. This often involves dietary modifications, lifestyle changes, and, in some cases, the use of medications or supplements to support histamine metabolism.

CHAPTER 3
Common Symptoms

3.1 Gastrointestinal Symptoms

Histamine intolerance commonly manifests with a range of gastrointestinal symptoms. These symptoms can vary in intensity and duration and often resemble those of other digestive conditions, making it challenging to diagnose. Some of the common gastrointestinal symptoms associated with histamine intolerance include:

1. **Abdominal Pain**: Many individuals with histamine intolerance experience abdominal pain, which can

range from mild discomfort to severe cramping.

2. **Bloating**: Excessive gas production and altered gut motility can lead to abdominal bloating, making the abdomen feel distended and uncomfortable.

3. **Diarrhea**: Histamine intolerance may result in episodes of diarrhea, characterized by loose, watery stools. This can be intermittent and is often triggered by ingesting high-histamine foods.

4. **Constipation**: On the flip side, some individuals may experience constipation, which can also be linked to histamine intolerance.

5. **Nausea**: Nausea and a feeling of queasiness are common gastrointestinal symptoms associated with histamine intolerance.

6. **Vomiting**: In more severe cases or during acute histamine reactions, vomiting may occur as the body attempts to rid itself of ingested histamine.

7. **Gastroesophageal Reflux (GERD)**: Histamine plays a role in gastric acid regulation, and individuals with histamine intolerance may experience symptoms of GERD, including heartburn and regurgitation.

8. **Irritable Bowel Syndrome (IBS)-like Symptoms**: Some of the gastrointestinal symptoms experienced in histamine

intolerance overlap with those of IBS, such as abdominal pain, diarrhea, and constipation.

These gastrointestinal symptoms can significantly impact an individual's quality of life, leading to discomfort and dietary restrictions.

3.2 Skin and Allergic Reactions

Histamine intolerance can also present with skin and allergic reactions, often mimicking the symptoms of allergies or dermatological conditions. Common skin and allergic reactions associated with histamine intolerance include:

1. **Hives (Urticaria)**: Hives are itchy, raised, red welts on the

skin. They can appear suddenly and may vary in size and shape.

2. **Pruritus (Itching)**: Persistent and generalized itching of the skin is a hallmark symptom of histamine intolerance.

3. **Redness (Erythema)**: The skin may become red or flushed, particularly in areas where hives or itching occur.

4. **Angioedema**: This is a deeper form of swelling that often affects the eyes, lips, and sometimes the throat. It can cause a sensation of tightness or difficulty breathing.

5. **Contact Dermatitis**: Some individuals with histamine intolerance may experience skin rashes or contact dermatitis as a result of

exposure to histamine-rich foods or substances that trigger histamine release.

6. **Flushing**: Histamine can dilate blood vessels, leading to flushing or a sensation of warmth in the skin.

7. **Runny Nose and Sneezing**: Histamine can cause nasal congestion, runny nose, and sneezing, similar to allergic rhinitis (hay fever) symptoms.

8. **Itchy or Watery Eyes**: Eye symptoms, including itching and excessive tearing, are common in histamine intolerance.

It's important to note that these skin and allergic reactions can occur suddenly and often in response to the ingestion of histamine-rich foods or the presence of other histamine-releasing factors. They can vary in severity and duration, and individuals with histamine intolerance may find themselves managing these symptoms on a regular basis. Recognizing these symptoms as potential indicators of histamine intolerance is a crucial step toward diagnosis and effective management.

3.3 Respiratory Symptoms

Histamine intolerance can extend its influence to the respiratory system, leading to various symptoms that can mimic those of respiratory allergies or asthma. These respiratory symptoms can range from mild to severe and may include:

1. **Coughing**: Individuals with histamine intolerance may experience persistent or intermittent coughing, similar to what is observed in allergic reactions or asthma.

2. **Wheezing**: Some people with histamine intolerance may develop wheezing, which is a high-pitched whistling sound when breathing, particularly during exhalation.

3. **Shortness of Breath**: Histamine-induced bronchoconstriction can cause a feeling of breathlessness or tightness in the chest.

4. **Chest Tightness**: Chest discomfort and tightness may occur, often due to the

constriction of airways and bronchial muscles.

5. **Nasal Congestion**: Histamine can lead to nasal congestion, which can result in difficulty breathing through the nose.

6. **Sneezing**: Individuals may experience increased episodes of sneezing, particularly when exposed to histamine-releasing substances or allergens.

7. **Postnasal Drip**: Excessive mucus production can result in postnasal drip, leading to throat irritation and coughing.

8. **Asthma-Like Symptoms**: Some individuals with histamine intolerance may exhibit symptoms resembling asthma, including coughing,

wheezing, and bronchial constriction.

These respiratory symptoms can be triggered by the presence of elevated histamine levels in the body, whether due to the consumption of histamine-rich foods or other factors that lead to histamine release. It's essential to recognize these symptoms as potential indicators of histamine intolerance, as they may be mistakenly attributed to other respiratory conditions. Accurate diagnosis and appropriate management can help alleviate these symptoms and improve respiratory health in affected individuals.

3.4 Other Systemic Symptoms

In addition to gastrointestinal, skin, allergic, and respiratory symptoms, histamine intolerance can lead to a wide range of other systemic symptoms. These symptoms can affect various parts of the body and can significantly impact an individual's overall well-being. Some of the common systemic symptoms associated with histamine intolerance include:

1. **Headaches and Migraines**: Histamine can dilate blood vessels in the brain, leading to headaches and, in some cases, severe migraines.

2. **Fatigue**: Many individuals with histamine intolerance report persistent fatigue, which may

be attributed to the chronic inflammation and discomfort caused by histamine-related symptoms.

3. **Dizziness and Lightheadedness**: These symptoms can result from histamine's effects on blood vessel dilation and low blood pressure.

4. **Cardiovascular Symptoms**: Some individuals may experience palpitations, irregular heartbeats, or changes in heart rate due to histamine's influence on the cardiovascular system.

5. **Joint Pain and Muscle Aches**: Histamine intolerance may cause joint pain and muscle aches, which can be mistaken

for other musculoskeletal
conditions.

6. **Mood Disturbances**:
Histamine's role in the brain
can lead to mood disturbances,
such as anxiety and irritability.

7. **Menstrual Irregularities**:
Some women may experience
changes in their menstrual
cycle and symptoms like
heavier or more painful periods
in association with histamine
intolerance.

8. **Sleep Disturbances**: Sleep
quality may be compromised,
with symptoms like difficulty
falling asleep, frequent
awakenings, or restless sleep.

9. **Throat and Vocal Cord
Symptoms**: Individuals may
experience throat discomfort, a

sensation of a lump in the throat, or changes in voice quality.

10. **Changes in Body Temperature**: Histamine can affect the body's thermoregulation, leading to sensations of heat, cold, or fluctuations in body temperature.

11. **Impaired Cognitive Function**: Some people with histamine intolerance may report brain fog, poor concentration, and difficulties with memory.

12. **Swelling (Edema)**: Swelling, particularly in the extremities, can occur due to histamine-induced changes in blood vessel permeability.

13.**Frequent Urination**: Increased urinary frequency may be observed as histamine affects the urinary system.

These systemic symptoms can be challenging to attribute to histamine intolerance, as they are not always directly associated with the digestive, skin, or respiratory systems. However, it's important to consider histamine intolerance as a potential underlying cause when experiencing a combination of these symptoms, especially if they worsen after consuming histamine-rich foods or in response to other triggers. Diagnosis and management tailored to the individual's needs can help alleviate these systemic symptoms and improve overall quality of life.

CHAPTER 4

Diagnosis and Testing

4.1 Medical History and Symptom Assessment

Diagnosing histamine intolerance often begins with a thorough medical history and symptom assessment. Healthcare providers rely on this initial step to gather information about the patient's health, lifestyle, and the nature of their symptoms. Here's how medical history and symptom assessment play a crucial role in diagnosing histamine intolerance:

1. Patient Interview: The healthcare provider will conduct a comprehensive interview to understand the patient's medical history, including any pre-existing conditions, allergies, and medications being taken. It's important for the patient to provide a detailed account of their symptoms, their onset, duration, and any potential triggers.

2. Dietary History: Information about the patient's diet is critical since histamine intolerance is often linked to the consumption of high-histamine foods and beverages. The healthcare provider may ask for a dietary history to identify any patterns related to symptom exacerbation after specific meals or dietary choices.

3. Symptom Assessment: The patient's description of symptoms is a key element in the diagnostic process. Symptoms associated with histamine intolerance can be diverse and may affect multiple systems, including the gastrointestinal, skin, respiratory, and other systems. The healthcare provider will inquire about specific symptoms, their frequency, and their impact on the patient's quality of life.

4. Onset and Timing: Identifying when symptoms occur and their temporal relationship to meals, stress, or other factors is crucial. Some individuals with histamine intolerance may notice a pattern of symptoms emerging shortly after consuming certain foods or beverages.

5. Duration and Progression: Understanding how long symptoms last and whether they have been progressive or consistent over time is important in assessing the severity and impact of histamine intolerance.

6. Response to Diet: The healthcare provider may ask about any dietary modifications the patient has made and whether these changes have had an effect on their symptoms. For instance, some individuals with histamine intolerance experience symptom relief on a low-histamine diet.

7. Triggers and Exacerbating Factors: Patients may be asked about specific triggers or situations that seem to worsen their symptoms. This can include stress, hormonal changes, alcohol consumption, and more.

8. Differential Diagnosis: The healthcare provider will consider other conditions with similar symptoms and rule them out. Conditions like food allergies, irritable bowel syndrome (IBS), and gastroesophageal reflux disease

(GERD) may have symptoms overlapping with histamine intolerance.

A comprehensive medical history and symptom assessment serve as the foundation for diagnosing histamine intolerance. While no single symptom or piece of information can definitively confirm the diagnosis, a detailed understanding of the patient's symptoms and their relationship to dietary and lifestyle factors is crucial for guiding further diagnostic tests and determining the most appropriate management strategies. It's also important for patients to be open and thorough in their communication with healthcare providers to ensure an accurate diagnosis.

4.2 Laboratory Tests

Laboratory tests can be valuable tools in the diagnosis of histamine intolerance, as they can provide supportive evidence of the condition. While there is no single definitive laboratory test for histamine intolerance, several tests can be performed to assess histamine levels and related factors:

a. Measurement of DAO Enzyme Activity: One of the key tests used to support the diagnosis of histamine intolerance is the measurement of diamine oxidase (DAO) enzyme activity. Low levels of DAO in the blood may suggest a deficiency in this enzyme, which is responsible for breaking down histamine. This test can help identify individuals with impaired histamine metabolism.

b. Measurement of Histamine Levels: Measuring histamine levels in the blood or urine can provide additional evidence of histamine intolerance. Elevated histamine levels may indicate that the body is not effectively metabolizing histamine.

c. Allergy Testing: Allergy tests, such as skin prick tests or blood tests for specific allergens, can help rule out true allergies as the cause of symptoms. It's important to differentiate between allergies and histamine intolerance, as the management and treatment strategies differ.

d. Comprehensive Stool Analysis: This test may be performed to assess the balance of gut microbiota and the presence of conditions like small intestinal bacterial overgrowth (SIBO) or other gastrointestinal issues that can contribute to histamine intolerance.

It's important to note that while these tests can provide valuable information, they are not standalone diagnostic tools. A diagnosis of histamine intolerance often relies on a combination of clinical evaluation, medical history, and the exclusion of other conditions with similar symptoms. Laboratory tests are used to support the diagnosis and confirm suspected histamine intolerance.

4.3 Elimination Diet

One of the most critical diagnostic tools for histamine intolerance is the elimination diet. This approach involves temporarily removing histamine-rich and histamine-releasing foods from the diet to see if symptoms improve. Here's how an elimination diet is typically conducted:

a. Preparation: Before starting the elimination diet, individuals are advised to keep a detailed food diary for a period, noting all foods and beverages consumed and the corresponding symptoms and their severity.

b. Elimination Phase: During the elimination phase, high-histamine foods and beverages are removed from the diet. This includes aged cheeses, fermented products, alcohol, processed meats, certain fruits and vegetables, and various other items known to be high in histamine. Some individuals may also need to avoid foods that can block DAO activity.

c. Symptom Monitoring:
Throughout the elimination phase, individuals should monitor their symptoms and their overall well-being. This helps track any improvements or changes that occur in response to the dietary modifications.

d. Reintroduction Phase: After a specified period (often a few weeks to a few months) of eliminating high-histamine foods, individual items are systematically reintroduced one at a time. During this phase, individuals monitor for the recurrence or worsening of symptoms, which can be a strong indicator of histamine intolerance if they occur after reintroducing specific foods.

The results of the elimination diet, in terms of symptom improvement and exacerbation upon reintroduction of certain foods, can be a crucial piece of evidence in diagnosing histamine intolerance. It helps identify specific dietary triggers and provides valuable insights into the condition. In some cases, healthcare providers may recommend conducting this diet under the guidance of a registered dietitian or nutritionist to ensure nutritional needs are met and that the process is systematic and controlled.

CHAPTER 5

Management and Treatment

5.1 Dietary Changes

Dietary modifications are a cornerstone of managing histamine intolerance. By making specific changes to your diet, you can reduce histamine intake and potentially alleviate many of the associated symptoms. Here are key dietary changes commonly recommended for managing histamine intolerance:

1. Low-Histamine Diet: Adopting a low-histamine diet is the primary dietary change for managing histamine intolerance. This involves avoiding or minimizing the consumption of foods that are naturally high in histamine or known to trigger histamine release. Some examples of high-histamine foods and beverages to limit or avoid include aged cheeses, processed meats, fermented foods, alcohol, and some fruits and vegetables. Instead, focus on fresh, unprocessed foods with lower histamine content.

2. Histamine-Free Diet: In severe cases or when symptom relief is not achieved with a low-histamine diet, some individuals may need to temporarily follow a histamine-free diet. This diet is more restrictive and eliminates even more high-histamine foods, aiming to reduce histamine intake to the minimum.

3. Monitor Food Freshness: Freshness matters in a histamine-restricted diet. opt for fresh foods over leftovers or items that have been stored for an extended period. Pay attention to expiration dates and food handling practices.

4. Food Preparation: Cooking methods can affect histamine levels in food. Grilling, frying, and roasting can increase histamine content, so consider steaming, boiling, or microwaving as cooking alternatives. Be cautious with the use of certain spices and seasonings, as some can contain histamine-releasing substances.

5. Avoid Certain Food Additives: Some food additives, such as monosodium glutamate (MSG) and sulfites, can trigger histamine release. Read food labels carefully to avoid these additives.

6. Gradual Reintroduction: After following a low-histamine or histamine-free diet for a period, work with a healthcare provider or dietitian to gradually reintroduce specific foods, one at a time. This helps identify individual triggers and determine which foods can be tolerated.

7. Keep a Food Diary: Maintaining a food diary can help you track your dietary choices and any associated symptoms. This can be particularly useful during the reintroduction phase, as it allows you to monitor your body's response to different foods.

8. Dietary Supplements: Some individuals with histamine intolerance may benefit from dietary supplements that support histamine metabolism. These can include DAO enzyme supplements or vitamin B6, which is involved in histamine degradation.

9. Stay Hydrated: Proper hydration can help flush excess histamine from the body. Drinking plenty of water can be especially important when experiencing symptoms.

10. Work with a Dietitian: Consider working with a registered dietitian or nutritionist experienced in histamine intolerance to ensure you are getting proper nutrition while adhering to dietary restrictions.

It's important to note that the severity of histamine intolerance varies from person to person, and not all individuals will require the same level of dietary restriction. The goal of dietary changes is to reduce histamine intake and identify specific triggers while still maintaining a balanced and nutritionally adequate diet. The guidance of a healthcare provider or dietitian is essential for creating a personalized dietary plan that suits your needs and helps manage histamine intolerance effectively.

5.2 Medications

While dietary changes are a fundamental component of managing histamine intolerance, medications can play a supportive role in alleviating symptoms and improving the quality of life for individuals with histamine intolerance. Here are some medications that may be considered as part of the treatment plan for histamine intolerance:

1. **Antihistamines:**
   Antihistamines are the most commonly used medications to

relieve the symptoms of histamine intolerance. They work by blocking histamine receptors in the body, reducing the effects of histamine. These are available both over-the-counter and as prescription medications. H1 antihistamines are often used to relieve allergy-like symptoms, while H2 antihistamines may help manage gastrointestinal symptoms like acid reflux.

2. **Proton Pump Inhibitors (PPIs):** In some cases, individuals with histamine intolerance may experience significant gastric acid production, leading to symptoms like acid reflux. Proton pump inhibitors, which reduce stomach acid

production, can be prescribed to alleviate these symptoms.

3. **Diamine Oxidase (DAO) Supplements:** DAO is the enzyme responsible for breaking down histamine in the digestive tract. In cases of a known or suspected DAO deficiency, supplements containing DAO can be taken before meals to support histamine metabolism. These supplements may help some individuals tolerate histamine-containing foods more effectively.

4. **Mast Cell Stabilizers:** Some medications, such as cromolyn sodium, work by stabilizing mast cells and preventing the release of histamine. These may be considered for individuals

with particularly severe symptoms.

5. **Leukotriene Modifiers:** Leukotrienes are inflammatory molecules that can work in conjunction with histamine to produce symptoms. Medications that modify leukotrienes, such as montelukast, may be used to manage respiratory and skin symptoms.

6. **Prescription Medications:** In some cases, healthcare providers may prescribe stronger antihistamines, corticosteroids, or other medications to manage severe symptoms during acute episodes.

It's important to note that the use of medications for histamine intolerance should be discussed with a healthcare provider, preferably one with experience in treating the condition. The choice of medication and the dosage will depend on the individual's specific symptoms and needs. In some instances, a combination of dietary changes and medication may provide the most effective symptom relief.

Additionally, medications can provide temporary relief, but the primary goal in managing histamine intolerance is to identify and address the underlying causes and triggers, which may involve dietary changes, lifestyle modifications, and addressing any underlying gastrointestinal issues. The use of medications is often part of a comprehensive approach to symptom management.

5.3 Lifestyle Modifications

In addition to dietary changes and medications, lifestyle modifications play a crucial role in managing histamine intolerance. These adjustments can help reduce symptom severity, minimize triggers, and improve overall well-being. Here are some important lifestyle modifications to consider:

1. Stress Management: Stress can exacerbate histamine intolerance symptoms, as it can trigger the release of histamine in the body. Engage in stress-reduction techniques such as mindfulness, deep breathing, yoga, meditation, and relaxation exercises. Regular physical activity can also help reduce stress.

2. Hormone Regulation: Hormonal fluctuations, especially in women, can influence histamine levels. Women may notice an increase in symptoms during their menstrual cycle. Discuss hormone management strategies with a healthcare provider, which may include hormonal birth control or other therapies.

3. Sleep Hygiene: Proper sleep is crucial for overall health and symptom management. Establish good sleep hygiene practices, such as maintaining a regular sleep schedule, creating a comfortable sleep environment, and avoiding stimulants like caffeine and electronic devices before bedtime.

4. Allergen Avoidance: Identify and avoid environmental allergens that can trigger histamine release, such as pollen, dust mites, and pet dander.

Using air purifiers and allergen-proof bedding may be helpful.

5. Smoking and Alcohol: Both smoking and alcohol consumption can exacerbate histamine intolerance symptoms. Quitting smoking and reducing or eliminating alcohol intake can lead to symptom improvement.

6. Hydration: Proper hydration can help flush excess histamine from the body. Ensure you drink enough water throughout the day.

7. Sun Exposure: Sunlight and heat can trigger histamine release, leading to symptoms like skin flushing. Avoid excessive sun exposure, use sunscreen, and wear appropriate clothing when outdoors in hot weather.

8. Avoid Overexertion: Physical exertion can lead to the release of histamine, so avoid overexertion, especially in hot or humid conditions. Engage in moderate exercise and monitor for symptom exacerbation.

9. Patient Education: Educate yourself about histamine intolerance, its causes, and its management. Understanding your condition can empower you to make informed decisions about your diet and lifestyle.

10. Social Support: Joining a support group or seeking support from friends and family can be helpful. Sharing your experiences and challenges with others who have histamine intolerance can provide emotional support and practical advice.

11. Food Label Reading: Develop the habit of reading food labels to identify potential sources of histamine and other triggering substances, such as food additives and preservatives. Understanding food labels can help you make informed food choices.

12. Regular Follow-Up: Continue to work with your healthcare provider to monitor your progress and make any necessary adjustments to your treatment plan. Regular follow-up appointments can help ensure that your symptoms are well-managed.

Lifestyle modifications are an integral part of managing histamine intolerance. While they may not directly address the underlying causes, they can significantly reduce the frequency and severity of symptoms, improving your overall quality of life. Combining dietary changes, medications, and lifestyle modifications provides a holistic approach to managing histamine intolerance effectively.

CHAPTER 6

Potential Complications

6.1 Nutritional Deficiencies

Histamine intolerance and the dietary restrictions it imposes can lead to potential nutritional deficiencies. Managing histamine intolerance often involves avoiding or limiting various high-histamine foods, which can reduce the intake of certain essential nutrients. Here are some potential nutritional deficiencies to be aware of and how to address them:

a. Vitamin B6 Deficiency: Vitamin B6 is essential for histamine metabolism. Individuals with histamine intolerance, particularly those following a strict histamine-free diet, may be at risk of vitamin B6 deficiency. To address this, consider vitamin B6 supplements under the guidance of a healthcare provider.

b. Calcium Deficiency: Dairy products are a common source of calcium, and many individuals with histamine intolerance avoid them due to their histamine content. To maintain adequate calcium intake, choose lactose-free or low-histamine dairy options or explore non-dairy calcium sources like fortified plant-based milk, leafy greens, and almonds.

c. Vitamin D Deficiency: Reduced dairy consumption and limited sun exposure (due to potential histamine release) can contribute to vitamin D deficiency. Consider vitamin D supplements or increase exposure to sunlight, with appropriate sun protection measures.

d. Iron Deficiency: Red meats are rich in iron, but histamine intolerance may limit their consumption. To prevent iron deficiency, consume other iron-rich foods like lean poultry, fish, legumes, and iron-fortified cereals. Combining iron-rich foods with sources of vitamin C can enhance iron absorption.

e. Fiber Deficiency: A low-histamine diet may reduce the intake of whole grains and certain high-fiber fruits and vegetables. Ensure you include fiber-rich options like quinoa, brown rice, and low-histamine fruits and vegetables to maintain healthy digestion.

f. Protein Intake: With dietary restrictions, individuals may need to be mindful of their protein intake. Select protein sources that are well-tolerated, such as lean poultry, eggs, fish, and low-histamine legumes.

g. Omega-3 Fatty Acids: Fish is a common source of omega-3 fatty acids, but its histamine content may limit its consumption. To maintain omega-3 intake, consider fish oil supplements or explore other sources like flaxseeds, chia seeds, and walnuts.

h. Micronutrients: Various vitamins and minerals found in a balanced diet can be affected by histamine intolerance and dietary restrictions. Regularly monitor your nutrient intake and consider working with a registered dietitian to ensure you are meeting your nutritional needs.

Supplements may be recommended in cases of documented deficiencies.

It's crucial to address potential nutritional deficiencies to prevent long-term health consequences. Consult with a healthcare provider or registered dietitian who can help you develop a well-balanced, histamine-friendly diet that meets your nutritional requirements. Additionally, regular monitoring of nutrient levels through blood tests can help identify and address deficiencies promptly.

6.2 Impact on Quality of Life

Histamine intolerance can have a significant impact on an individual's quality of life. While it is not a life-threatening condition, the chronic nature of the symptoms and the need for dietary and lifestyle modifications can affect various aspects of daily living. Here are some ways in which histamine intolerance can influence quality of life:

1. Dietary Limitations: Following a low-histamine or histamine-free diet can be challenging, as it involves avoiding many common and enjoyable foods. This restriction can lead to frustration and feelings of deprivation, affecting the pleasure of eating.

2. Social and Recreational Activities: Dining out, attending social gatherings, or enjoying recreational activities that involve food can become more complicated. Social interactions may be impacted, as explaining dietary restrictions to others can be difficult.

3. Emotional Well-being: The chronic nature of histamine intolerance and its symptoms can lead to emotional distress, including stress, anxiety, and depression. Dealing with persistent symptoms and the uncertainty of when they might occur can be emotionally taxing.

4. Sleep Disruption: Histamine intolerance can lead to sleep disturbances, as symptoms like itching, flushing, and digestive discomfort can interfere with a good night's sleep. Poor sleep can have a cascading effect on overall well-being.

5. Work and Productivity: Symptoms can affect work performance and productivity.

Gastrointestinal symptoms, headaches, and fatigue can make it challenging to concentrate and be productive, potentially impacting career and income.

6. Physical and Mental Fatigue: The energy expended in managing dietary choices, monitoring symptoms, and seeking solutions can lead to physical and mental fatigue, affecting the overall quality of life.

7. Relationship Strain: Living with histamine intolerance can place strain on personal relationships, as partners, family, and friends may need to adjust their routines and meals to accommodate dietary restrictions.

8. Healthcare Costs: The need for medical consultations, dietary supplements, and potential prescription medications can result in increased healthcare costs, which can be a financial burden.

9. Impact on Travel: Traveling can be more challenging due to the need to adhere to dietary restrictions and navigate unfamiliar food options. Planning and preparation are essential when traveling with histamine intolerance.

10. Limited Exercise and Physical Activity: Some individuals may avoid physical activity due to concerns about symptom exacerbation or overexertion. This can impact overall fitness and well-being.

11. Body Image and Self-esteem: Skin-related symptoms like hives, itching, and flushing can impact body image and self-esteem, affecting self-confidence and self-worth.

It's important to recognize the psychosocial impact of histamine intolerance and its potential to affect quality of life. Seeking support from healthcare providers, dietitians, and support groups can be valuable in managing the condition and addressing the emotional and social challenges it presents. Additionally, finding effective symptom management strategies can help individuals with histamine intolerance regain a sense of control over their lives and improve their overall well-being.

CHAPTER 7
Coping Strategies

7.1 Support and Resources

Coping with histamine intolerance can be challenging, but there are various sources of support and resources available to help individuals navigate this condition effectively. Here are some valuable sources of support:

a. Healthcare Providers: Consult with healthcare professionals, such as allergists, gastroenterologists, dietitians, and nutritionists, who have experience in managing histamine intolerance. They can provide guidance on diagnosis, treatment, and dietary planning.

b. Registered Dietitians: Work with a registered dietitian who specializes in histamine intolerance. They can create personalized meal plans and provide guidance on safe food choices and nutrient supplementation.

c. Support Groups: Joining a support group or online community of individuals dealing with histamine intolerance can provide emotional support, practical advice, and a sense of belonging. Sharing experiences and tips with others who understand the challenges can be highly beneficial.

d. Online Resources: There are numerous websites, forums, and social media groups dedicated to histamine intolerance. These platforms often offer a wealth of information, including dietary guidelines, recipes, and personal experiences.

e. Educational Materials: Seek out books, articles, and research papers on histamine intolerance to deepen your understanding of the condition, its causes, and management strategies.

f. Mental Health Support: If you are experiencing emotional distress, consider seeking support from a mental health professional. Therapy or counseling can help you manage the emotional impact of living with histamine intolerance.

7.2 Strategies for Living with Histamine Intolerance

Living with histamine intolerance requires a proactive approach and various coping strategies to manage symptoms and maintain a good quality of life. Here are some strategies for effectively living with histamine intolerance:

a. Food Preparation and Planning:

- Carefully plan your meals to ensure they are low in histamine or adhere to your specific dietary restrictions.

- Batch-cook and freeze histamine-friendly meals for convenience.

- Consider investing in kitchen appliances like a slow cooker or pressure cooker to simplify cooking.

b. Food Label Reading:

- Develop the habit of reading food labels to identify potential sources of histamine, allergens, and food additives.

- Familiarize yourself with common high-histamine foods and ingredients to avoid surprises.

c. Symptom Tracking:

- Keep a symptom journal to track the foods you eat and any symptom patterns. This can help you identify specific triggers and adjust your diet accordingly.

d. Gradual Reintroduction:

- Work with a healthcare provider or dietitian to systematically reintroduce foods after an elimination diet. This can help identify safe and tolerated foods.

e. Stress Management:

- Implement stress-reduction techniques like mindfulness, meditation, deep breathing, or yoga to minimize the emotional and physical impact of stress.

f. Social Support:

- Communicate with friends and family about your dietary restrictions and educate them about histamine intolerance to ease social interactions.

g. Medication Management:

- Take prescribed medications as directed by your healthcare provider to manage symptoms effectively.

h. Supplements:

- If necessary, consider dietary supplements to address potential nutritional deficiencies, but only under the guidance of a healthcare provider.

i. Lifestyle Adjustments:

- Make necessary lifestyle changes to accommodate histamine intolerance, such as modifying exercise routines or travel plans.

j. Patience and Self-care:

- Be patient with yourself and practice self-compassion.

Living with histamine intolerance can be challenging, but it's important to prioritize self-care and self-acceptance.

k. Monitor Your Health:

- Regularly consult with your healthcare provider to monitor your health, evaluate treatment effectiveness, and address any new symptoms or concerns.

Histamine intolerance may present challenges, but with the right support, resources, and coping strategies, individuals can effectively manage their symptoms and enjoy an improved quality of life. The key is to take a proactive and well-informed approach to address this condition and its impact on daily living.